The Athletic Scholarship Myth

Why Year-Round Youth Sports are a Prescription for Failure

Dr. Robert E. Berry

Board Certified Orthopedic Surgeon
Fellowship Trained in Sports Medicine

The Athletic Scholarship Myth

Printed by:
CreateSpace Independent
Publishing Platform

Copyright © 2017, Dr. Robert E. Berry

Published in the United States of America

Book ID: 160526-00431

ISBN-13: 978-1546312048
ISBN-10: 1546312048

No parts of this publication may be reproduced without correct attribution to the author of this book.

Here's What's Inside...

Introduction 1

The Way It Used to Be 3

Burnout 7

Traditional Strength-Training Programs
Lead to Decreased Athletic Performance
and Increased Injuries 13

Elbow Injuries 18

Knee Injuries 23

Head Injuries 24

Sports Performance Centers 29

Friday Night Lights 35

Psych Issues: Anxiety and Depression 44

Regulating Sports 47

Select Snobs 55

Choosing to Play Just One Sport 63

The Sandlot: Where Did It Go? 66

"Show Me the Money!" 68

Coaches and Training Techniques 72

Heat and Hydration 73

When Did Cheerleading Become Competitive Gymnastics?.. 81

Self-Confidence vs. Self-Esteem 83

Are Kids Really Better Today?.................................. 85

How to Get the Same Level of Care as Professional Athletes 87

Dedication

To my wife Christy, who married me when I was 19 years old bagging groceries, but always believed I was capable of more.

To my children Mark, Kylie and Blake who have taught me more about life than they know and resisted the pressure of playing year round sports.

To my grandfather who raised me and drove 200 miles a day for work and still took me to my practices every night and on weekends.

To my grandmother, who left this world far too soon, raised me like her son and was my biggest fan. When doctors thought I had ADHD at 5 and wanted to put me on medication, my grandmother said no and enrolled me in soccer. You might say sports, were my own therapy early in life. As I excelled in sports in high school, setting school records in the 400m, I will forever hear my grandmother's cheers as I rounded the last corner and headed home...
"Go Robert!" I have never looked back.

Introduction

As a father of three—two boys who participated in sports growing up and had their share of injuries, along with a daughter who participated in competitive gymnastics and cheer—I understand the desire and pressure for your child to have all of the opportunities afforded to them by playing sports competitively. However, as an orthopedic surgeon also trained in sports medicine, who spent a career taking care of professional athletes as well as athletes of all ages, shapes, and sizes, I've seen an epidemic of injuries in young athletes over the last several years.

My role is not only to treat the patients and the injuries that present themselves in my clinic, but also to help educate parents to prevent them in the first place. It's become increasingly important to educate coaches, parents, and the athletes themselves on the things they do that put them at risk for injuries. This book is my way of coaching, if you will, these individuals on what they can do to prevent further injuries.

I feel it's time for someone to be a champion and to step up for the young athletes—our children—and educate them on what is really going on when they play sports year-round and why we are seeing such a rampant increase in preventable injuries that often have lifelong ramifications.

Enjoy the book!

I hope this book encourages you to allow your child to be a kid and enjoy sports, instead of seeing it as a job with the hope of a future scholarship, which statistically will never come. I also hope this book educates you on why year-round youth sports are a prescription for failure and why sports specialization is so dangerous.

To Your Success!

Robert E. Berry, DO

The Way It Used to Be

Whatever happened to kids just having fun? When I was growing up, kids played sports because they were fun. We didn't have personal trainers; we had coaches. Most of us grew up playing local Little League, football, soccer, volleyball, and other sports, and most of us played sports because we enjoyed them. It gave us time away with friends and allowed us to burn off unused energy pent up from sitting in school all day.

I can remember running home from school and gathering with friends at the end of the street for a pickup game of baseball or football. It was a simpler time back then, and summer days seemed to last forever. Kids didn't go to sports performance training or personal position coaches; they simply went outside with friends and played whatever sports they could.

Somewhere along the way, youth sports went very wrong. By the time kids are nine or ten, they are told that they have to pick which individual sport they're going to play. Child athletes are told by coaches and sometimes parents that they must focus on one sport, or they won't be good enough to play in high school or beyond. Children are told by some coaches and well-meaning parents that if they ever want to have a chance of lettering in a sport or have hopes of playing college sports, they have to choose now and commit. Instead of after-school pickup games, it's off to mini-camps, after-school sports, personal position coaches, and sports performance training programs. The motto seems to be, "You can never start too young."

When children get home in the evenings, they scramble to finish whatever homework they have. They become multi-taskers early on, studying at the dinner table while shoveling food into their mouths. With all of the homework piled on kids these days, they usually go to bed late, wake up tired, and do it all over again. No wonder so many kids take energy drinks just to keep going.

This vicious cycle starts in the early to later elementary years. By the time the child reaches high school, they are burned out on sports and tired of having no life. Promising athletes hang it up before they really get started. It's a shame that sports, which used to be a stress-reliever, has become a stress-producer.

As an orthopedic surgeon specializing in sports medicine, I have seen an alarming increase in the number of injuries in young children. Even during my training, I never saw the amount of injuries I witness today. The sad thing is that most of the injuries are the results of overtraining or too much, too soon.

It's alarming to think that so many of the children I see in my practice, who started out loving their sports, end up burned out or injured. The years of year-round training, offseason sports performance, and personal position coaching take their toll.

Some of the greatest athletes that I have had the opportunity to work with from the NFL, soccer, hockey, rugby, cycling, etc. never even played competitive sports until they were freshmen in high school. A great example is Drew Brees, Super Bowl MVP and quarterback of the World Champion New Orleans Saints. Drew didn't play football until he was a freshman at Westlake High school in Austin, Texas. Growing up he played sports with friends or his older brother, which is when he formed his competitive spirit.

I worked with Drew from 2004 to 2005, while I was with the San Diego Chargers. He is one of the most competitive individuals and one of the nicest, but he didn't grow up with a personal position coach or at an after-school sports performance center.

Football players often say that a body can only take so many "hits." I think delaying the punishment of contact sports, like football, is a wise choice. It is mind boggling to me that parents and coaches tell children that if they want to have a chance to play in high school or college, they have to start planning their futures when they're nine or ten years old.

If the goal is to allow children to excel in sports and be able to play in high school or college, we should take a lesson from those who really are the best at their games. What did the professional athletes do to get where they are? Did they start playing their sports at young ages? Did they have personal trainers or nutritionists as children? Did they have personal performance training coaches at nine or ten years of age? Did they have to choose between many sports that they enjoyed playing as youths to focus on one sport in late elementary school or junior high?

If the answers are "no," then why are we making our kids do this? Well-meaning parents have bought into the fear tactics of some coaches and sports performance training programs. If most professional players didn't do it to get where they are, why are we making sports a job for kids? They only get to be kids once. Sports should be fun, and we as parents must make sure that it's about the kids and not about us.

Burnout

It seems that kids get burned out on sports before they even have an opportunity to get started. Kids who have participated in year-round youth sports from early childhood want nothing to do with them by the time they get to high school. It's not uncommon in my practice to see kids who "fake" injuries, so they don't have to play anymore.

A friend of mine cares for elite gymnasts and is often consulted as a last resort for strange complaints and injuries that have never received definitive diagnoses by other doctors. This physician tells me that often he separates the child from the parents and questions them privately. Sometimes the child breaks down in tears when interviewed away from the parents about their "injury." The child may say that they don't really have an injury but that they don't know how to tell their parents that despite all of the financial sacrifices made for them to get where they are, the child doesn't want to do it anymore. Sometimes the child hopes that the doctor will be the bad guy and tell the parents that the child has a career-ending injury and can't continue on. The child doesn't have the courage to confront their parents and simply say that they are finished. It's a sad thing to see.

A family friend of mine had a daughter who was an elite ice skater. She was on track to be in the Olympics. Unfortunately, she hit puberty, began to develop, and gained weight. She couldn't perform the jumps and spins that once came effortlessly. Her family had sold their home and lived in a small apartment with the other two children so their daughter could be near the ice rink. Her family homeschooled her, and ice skating consumed her. She was up at 5 AM and trained for hours on end.

Unfortunately, she suffered a significant hip injury. Despite surgery, she was unable to return to the sport she loved. Her Olympic aspirations were gone, and she went on a downward spiral of drugs and alcohol, all before she could even drive. The family was devastated, and dreams were never realized. I wish this story were rare, but it is all too common in the world of elite youth sports.

If the goal is to allow a child to play a sport for fun, or for the possibility of playing in high school, college, and beyond, shouldn't we try to protect them, so they are able to perform when it really matters? It's important to look at the professional athletes whom our children have as heroes and examples. Many of these athletes, with whom I've worked on a professional level, never even played competitive football or baseball until they were freshmen in high school or beyond. I believe this allowed them to keep the sport fresh and exciting and to be able to peak at the right times. Children with bodies that aren't developed have a difficult time performing at high levels and may peak too early and become burned out, never having a chance to realize their dreams.

It is now common for children in school who want to play one sport to participate in additional sports at the requirements of their coaches. For instance, someone who desires to play football may be required to participate in offseason weightlifting/powerlifting programs in addition to being on the track team. All of these activities require their own practice schedules and commitments before school, after school, and on weekends. For a young adolescent, this can become overwhelming. Soon, just wanting to play football is not fun, but a full-time job.

Coaches play one athlete against another. If someone is injured, coaches may make fun of them and dismiss their injury as "faking it," saying that if they can't make off-season, "voluntary" practice, they shouldn't expect to play during the regular season. Not only do the athletes get burned out by these levels of activity, but their parents do as well.

We have bought into the lie that in order to be good at something, we need to do more of it.

There is a thing in sports medicine known as "overtraining." All of us who are familiar with taking care of athletes are aware that athletes need time to heal, to rest, and to recover in order to improve their levels of performance. Most would agree that it is not wise to lift the same amount of weight and train the same body part day after day without giving the body a rest period, but this is exactly what we do to our young athletes. We require them to participate in football; to lift weights before school; and to then participate in track, during which they run, sprint, and lift weights again.

Children who may like to play baseball and football can find themselves playing up to three or four sports at once. If a child refuses to participate in track or powerlifting, for instance, they will be ridiculed by the coaches at times, pressured, and often flat-out told that they will not play on the school team unless they perform in the so-called "elective" programs. While usually I am not one to encourage government involvement at the local level, I think that we have reached an epidemic of burnout and believe that something has to be done to protect our children. I do not believe that the coaches are capable of protecting our children.

There needs to be some sort of regulation for youth sports, from middle school and beyond, that clearly states when children can practice, which coaches are able to participate in these practices, and abolishing so-called elective training programs. All of us who have participated in these elective training programs realize that they are not so elective and that roll is being taken. Certainly the other student athletes and coaches know who is there, and that definitely affects who plays and participates, which is not fair. The only way to balance the scale is to eliminate these offseason elective programs.

When I was growing up, you could easily letter in three varsity sports; football, soccer, and track, for instance. All of these had different seasons, and it was understood by coaches and players that when you completed one sport, you simply moved to the next. The athlete who was a football player as well as a baseball player did not need to start offseason football training as well. I see too many kids who fall asleep in school; have unexplained aches and pains; and feel extreme pressure, stress, and clinical depression, all because they want to be able to play sports.

I think it is time that we do our best as parents, as coaches, and as physicians to protect our young children from burnout. We have gone from the extreme of competitive sports to indoctrinating our children with the idea that by age nine or ten, they must pick the one sport that they want to play for the rest of their lives and then participate in year-round training to achieve a level of high performance. I think this decision has been catastrophic, and many young, great athletes will never have the opportunity to realize their dreams because they simply get burned out. All of us who care for children—parents, coaches, and physicians—must step back and reevaluate why our kids play sports to begin with.

Sports are supposed to be fun. They're supposed to be a distraction from the rigors of academia. It is important to have a balance between body, mind, and spirit, but when all of the focus becomes the body, the other areas become unbalanced. I think it is crucial for our children that we acknowledge this imbalance and begin to make changes. After all, kids are only kids once.

Traditional Strength-Training Programs Lead to Decreased Athletic Performance and Increased Injuries

This title alone is controversial enough for traditional coaches and athletes. Most have been told that if they want to be faster and stronger, they need to lift more weights and do more squats. Recent research has shown that the traditional programs that athletes have done for years don't improve athletic performance and may actually hinder athletic performance.

Lance Walker is Director of Sports Performance for the Michael Johnson Center in McKinney, Texas. The Michael Johnson Center has gained national recognition as one of the premiere locations for elite athletes to train. Often, the people who train our youth and athletes in how to perform these lifts have done them wrong themselves for years and have never been properly instructed on how to perform them, so the cycle perpetuates itself.

If the objective of sports performance training is to create stronger, more flexible, and ultimately better athletes, then it seems we should have, as we do in medicine, performance outcome measures to determine what really works. We need to ask what really works and what is effective in helping our athletes not only become stronger and faster, but healthier and more resistant to athletic injuries. For years, I can recall football coaches saying that if you want to be faster and more explosive, you have to squat more. We found in recent years that squats not only lead to knee injuries, but can actually lead to slower athletes.

If done incorrectly, squats can build a quadriceps-dominant athlete, in which the front of the thigh is much stronger than the back of the thigh. This muscle imbalance is often perpetuated as an athlete ages from early adolescence into high school and college, leading to an increase in anterior cruciate ligament injuries and chronic hamstring injuries because the front of the leg overpowers the back of the leg. Squats have been almost a religion in football. If a football player refused to do squats or traditional powerlifts, the old-school coaches and even some new coaches trained under the old philosophy believed that they couldn't build speed and strength, but what is the NFL doing? What are the professional athletes doing?

One of the greatest athletes that I had the opportunity to work with is LaDainian Tomlinson (LT). A previous NFL MVP and arguably one of the greatest running backs to have ever played the game, he has a very atypical training program.

Although the specifics of B. Tomlinson's training program are kept under wraps, I can tell you from personal experience that it doesn't include the traditional lifts that are done in high schools and colleges around the United States.

My friend Todd Durkin, Director of Fitness 10 in San Diego, CA, has trained LT for many years. Todd's training programs are quite unique, as his list of professional athletes will tell you. The programs are athlete and sport-specific. Instead of having athletes do traditional powerlifts, which do not improve athletic performance, his programs center around core activities.

I think it is important for us to evaluate the strength and conditioning programs that we make our athletes undergo and ask the key question: Are these effective? If the things that we require athletes to do are not effective, then we should eliminate them.

The early 1960s Chargers and other football teams didn't encourage weightlifting. They believed that simply lifting weights would make you big, bulky, and less mobile, thereby making you less "athletic." The San Diego Chargers were one of the first teams to hire a strength and conditioning coach. That was the start of what we know today as traditional weight-training programs in football and athletics. However, as stated above, some of these traditional powerlifts have become almost a rite of passage—a religion of a sort—and do not necessarily improve athletes' performances.

An "I-had-to-do-it-so-you-have-to-do-it" philosophy exists, even if it's been proven to actually hurt athletes or inhibit athletic performance. In medicine we realized that just because our predecessors did it, doesn't mean it was the best way to train physicians.

It was not uncommon for resident physicians in training to work 100 or more hours per week and sometimes more in surgical specialties. Several years ago a group of physicians in New York challenged this notion of working residents until they drop. These young physicians were instrumental in new regulations that limit the number of hours resident physicians can work to 80 hours. It was found that when residents and doctors in training worked beyond time limits, their performances were less than those of well-rested physicians, and their judgments could be less than stellar. This fatigue was felt to lead to errors that could put patients' safety at risk. As a surgeon myself, I worked many 100-hour weeks and stayed up for several days at a time. While I recall being tired, I don't feel I ever put a patient's safety at risk. I personally felt that the longer hours were necessary to provide patient continuity and to provide young surgeons with exposure to pathology and experience.

Medicine has moved on to be performance-based and measure outcomes. Insurance companies now require groups of physicians to practice according to sets of guidelines, or not get paid. The idea is that these outcome-based guidelines lead to better outcomes and improved patient care.

This same philosophy needs to be applied to sports performance and conditioning, with the end goal in mind. If the goal is to create faster, stronger, better-performing athletes, then we should devise and develop exercise programs that produce these results in athletes. Simply telling athletes that because I did it, you have to is irrational and does not accomplish the end goal. We all know the definition of insanity: doing the same thing and expecting different results.

Elbow Injuries

Elbow injuries are one of the injuries I see most in young, skeletally immature baseball players. On a weekly basis I see otherwise healthy baseball players whose parents believe that they will be the next Nolan Ryan or Cliff Lee. These parents allow their children to not only pitch at very young ages, but to play baseball year-round. Even though there are guidelines and regulations for pitch counts per game, coaches and parents often ignore them. When the game is on the line, it seems to be okay to sacrifice a young athlete's elbow for the sake of winning.

I believe that the most dangerous thing for many young pitchers is to be too good, too soon. These young, talented pitchers get picked up by select teams and used up by some coaches with big egos or dads who are living through their kids. I can hardly contain myself when parents bring their young pitchers in to see me and say, "We just want whatever is best for Johnny" and, without a pause, finish the statement by saying, "When will he be back?" Often my job is to protect kids from their coaches or their parents. The very people who should be looking out for them often have their own agendas. The agenda of coaches is to win games and further their careers. For parents, it is often to get their children scholarships. One thing is for sure in sports medicine: The injuries are often the easiest things to take care of; dealing with coaches and parents is the most difficult.

The immature elbow has several growth plates. These growth plates appear around one year of age and fuse by the time the child is 14 years of age. If they over-stress the elbow during this growth phase, the growth plates can become injured and cause the elbow to be painful and grow crooked. If the elbow is put at rest when pain occurs, it will often heal itself. If, however, an athlete continues to throw in pain, irreversible damage can occur. The elbow experiences most of its development right in the middle of those Little League years. This is why it is so critical to adhere to pitch counts and not allow an athlete who is in pain to throw.

Recently, an 11-year-old came into my practice who was an excellent baseball player. He was allowed to pitch several times per week, and he pitched year-round. At times, he had been allowed to throw up to 80 or 90 pitches in a game, which is a pitch count almost twice what is recommended by orthopedic surgeons and physicians. This young athlete will likely never be able to play baseball again; certainly, he'll never be able to return to pitching. Sadly, all of that could have been prevented.

One of the hardest things that I have to face as an orthopedic sports medicine specialist is telling young athletes—or parents—that they will likely never play or participate again. Often this information or recommendation is met with resistance and sometimes hostility from the parents. Parents and coaches do not want to believe the facts. It is this same philosophy and attitude that gets their young children/athletes into these very situations.

Parents often leave my office upset and then seek out many other physicians in the hopes that they will be told something different. They seek out someone who will tell them what they want to hear. Sometimes these parents find physicians who have less training or experience in the field of sports medicine. Once they hear what they want to hear, or a physician suggests that their children may be able to return more quickly, they label the other doctors "quacks." I offer many second opinions on athletes, and my radar goes off when a parent speaks badly about another physician. All of us in medicine realize that if we don't tell them what they want to hear, these same parents will speak badly about us when they leave our offices.

I am okay with this, and I think anyone who cares for athletes, especially children, must be okay with it as well. My job is to do what is best for the athlete, not to tell someone what they want to hear. If I catered to parents and coaches instead of doing what is right, word would get around, and I would ultimately lose the respect of my colleagues. I often tell parents and coaches who don't like what I have to say to get another opinion and give them names of trusted colleagues. As a parent myself, I want what is best for the kids.

One of my common speeches is about elbow injuries in young pitchers. I often tell my patients and their families that a child's elbow is the only one that God gave them and the only one they will have for the rest of their life. I go on to explain that it is my job to protect them and to make sure that they have a healthy body that will allow them to live life and do work. Not every young Little Leaguer will make it to the major leagues, and certainly no one that has a bum elbow will.

I discuss "pitch counts" with patients, parents, and coaches, as well as types of pitches. Young pitchers may adhere to pitch counts but are allowed to throw curves or breaking balls too soon. Even the wrong kind of pitch thrown under a pitch count can injure an elbow. There are certain types of "curveballs" that can be thrown more like a football—so the wrist is not snapped—and that produce less force on the elbow and prevent devastating injuries. Unfortunately, these curves do not produce the same level of breaking, so these young pitchers still snap their wrists and throw curves well before it is recommended.

This early adoption of curves and breaking balls leads to severe stress on skeletally immature elbows and leads to devastating and potentially career-ending injuries. I have seen a disturbing increase in the number of ulnar collateral ligament sprains, which often lead to the "Tommy John" surgery. These injuries can be prevented by adhering to simple guidelines on throwing. What our grandmothers told us is true in sports medicine: "A pound of prevention is worth a ton of cure."

Knee Injuries

I have seen an increased number of knee injuries in recent years. The number of young female soccer players sustaining anterior cruciate ligaments is staggering. Often, these females are already at risk because of anatomical variations in knee injuries, but because of the increased number of teams on which they play, their risk is further increased. Often, these same children do workouts at school in middle school and high school, including squats and powerlifting, at a young age. This leads to the quadriceps-dominant athletes referenced above. These athletes sometimes have to have several knee surgeries before even leaving high school. Needless to say, these early knee injuries predispose these young athletes to developing debilitating arthritis in later years, which may ultimately require knee replacements.

Head Injuries

Head injuries are one of the most devastating things that we see in sports medicine. Sadly, guidelines have shown that closed head injuries or concussions are likely under-diagnosed and often mismanaged. Previously we had felt that if an athlete was simply "dazed" but returned to his normal state, he could return to play. If an athlete was able to perform exertional maneuvers on the sidelines and answer a battery of questions appropriately, it was felt that he could safely return to the event without fear of significant ill effects. Recent data supports that these athletes should be held back from contact for at least a week, sometimes longer. We are just now beginning to understand the long-term effects of closed head injuries or concussions. Long-term studies are happening now to understand the effects of repeated closed head injuries in contact sports.

We also know that in younger athletes, because of the disproportionate size of the head in relationship to the body, the neck is often not strong enough to support the head, which leads to further stress on the neck and spine. Children that are not appropriately instructed in youth sports and tackling may have associated neck injuries as well.

It is scary to me as a physician to realize that often the first line of evaluation treatment is well-meaning coaches who receive absolutely no training in the management of head or neck injuries in collision sports, such as hockey, football, and even soccer. I have gotten into arguments with coaches and even paramedics and medical personnel who are probably well-meaning but simply not educated in the management of head and neck injuries.

These individuals sometimes feel that if they say that little Johnny or Sally are okay, somehow they are. Living in the time of outcome-based medicine, it doesn't matter what one thinks; it matters what the evidence says. All of us need to begin to follow the guidelines and regulations established by our medical experts in order to protect our young athletes from permanent disabilities. Moving an athlete who has sustained a closed head injury or potential neck injury can be devastating, and there are no second chances. I have witnessed drills in which an athlete who is being punished is allowed to be hit by the entire team while going through two lines of players, shoulder-to-shoulder. I can recall a very large athlete who was being punished for his lack of performance on the field and was put through the so-called "gauntlet" drill. As I watched this child go through the line and be hit by the first two or three players, I noticed that he seemed to become wobbly on his feet and unstable. He was then hit by another group of two players in the line and immediately went down. The player was unresponsive.

I immediately went to his aid. I notified surrounding people to call 9-1-1 and, giving them some basic instruction, began to administer the care that I could to him on the field. The poor child was not able to move his arms or legs, and when he came to, it was clear that he had at least sustained a concussion. He was confused, dazed, and could not even tell me his name. This was one of the scariest situations that I have been involved with, but it only got worse.

Once the paramedics arrived, they began to attempt to remove his helmet and shoulder pads, which is highly discouraged when dealing with potential closed head injuries or cervical spine injuries. This child could hardly move his arms or legs and definitely had clinical evidence of a closed head injury and a cervical spine injury, and paramedics attempted to remove his helmet.

I instructed the paramedics that this was not protocol. I notified their base station, a local hospital from which they receive their instructions, that there was a surgeon on-site, providing care. You would assume that these paramedics would want to do what was best for the child, but I have often found that paramedical personnel turn these situations into turf battles. Egos get in the way of trying to do what is right and appropriate for patients.

In this particular case, even a respiratory therapist and other people tried to tell me to let the paramedics do their jobs, but if the paramedics had removed the child's helmet and shoulder pads, they could have caused a devastating injury and made the child a quadriplegic for the rest of their life, if not killed him.

With negotiation and by assuming control of the scene, which is something that a trained physician can do, we were able to properly immobilize the patient and get him to the children's trauma center, where it was confirmed that he did have a cervical spine injury and a closed head injury. To this day, this child—now nearly 18 years old—has never played football again and likely never will.

This case represents something that happens in America every day. The scary thing is that this incidence occurred in one of the largest cities in southern California, where you would expect to find highly trained medical personnel. This particular instance led to a city- and county-wide training program to re-educate paramedics and paramedical personnel on the evaluation and treatment of head and neck injuries in athletes.

Fortunately for this child, he lived. He is living an otherwise healthy life, although he never was able to return to the sport that he loved.

It is hard to know whether or not this child would have sustained this injury had his coaches not tried to punish him by allowing the entire team to take shots at him, which ultimately led to his injury. Certainly injuries can occur on the fields of competitive sports, but it does seem to me that our coaches and parents, in whom we instill our trust to care for our children, should not be using these types of punishments, which can have devastating consequence.

Sports Performance Centers

When I was growing up, sports performance centers were unheard of. Coaches volunteered their time to show young athletes how to properly play particular sports. Often, these coaches did not have any special training but hearts and love for the sports they were involved with. Many of these coaches had played sports themselves as youth or in high school and college, and some had even participated at the semi-pro or professional levels; however, it is not common for many of our youth coaches to have specialized training in athletic performance or in particular areas of sport.

A dad who played baseball at a high level and was a great outfielder or shortstop but has never pitched before, may have a difficult time instructing a young pitcher in proper form and technique. Proper form and technique for pitching is vitally important because it can be very influential when it comes to the development of elbow injuries, especially in young pitchers.

A recent research study done in a children's hospital in San Diego, California revealed that there is actually an ideal pitching form. We know from this research that when you train a pitcher to pitch more like this ideal form, the stress on their elbow and shoulder is much less, and their velocity and accuracy improve.

Having a specialty coach who instructs young athletes or pitchers on proper form and technique is a good thing. Young football players who want to be good quarterbacks need specialty instruction in this area, much like a baseball player, to protect their shoulders and elbows and to become more accurate. As competitiveness in youth sports has increased, so has the need to gain an edge. This is why I believe specialty coaches in sports performance centers have popped up everywhere around the United States. Parents who want their kids to have an edge and to be able to play varsity sports in high school or to play in college or professionally want to give their kids any possible advantage over the competition.

While I believe that the majority of parents are well-meaning, it can become a vicious cycle. What starts off as simple instruction on pitching turns into subsequent training and drills on plyometrics and core strengthening. While these are all good things, they begin to suck the time away from already busy youngsters. Many coaches run their own businesses, which have overhead to meet. They recommend further lessons and more subspecialty training in a particular area of sport. This subspecialty training requires more lessons and more money spent by the parents. This is quite a task when you have just one child, but if you have a family of two or three, or even more, it becomes a full-time job for one person to run the kids around to these specialty performance training centers in addition to their regular games and practices.

One of the fundamental principles of sports performance is proper rest and nutrition. With so many activities scheduled for children, this basic principle is often sacrificed. Kids are picked up from school often by a friend or family member; rushed through a fast-food restaurant; and while gobbling down their food on the way to practice, attempting to do homework in the car. These kids may not get home until 9:00 or 10:00 at night, they still have to finish their homework, and we wonder why they are tired in school.

After having worked with thousands of young athletes and many professional athletes, there is something to be said for genetic advantage. Some kids are just born natural athletes. I'm not saying that someone who works hard cannot improve their athletic ability or give themselves a slight edge, but I do believe that these people are few and far between. Sports performance centers, while well-meaning, have at times given a level of false hope to young athletes. These athletes believe, as do their parents, that if they just attend enough performance-training sessions and specialty coaching clinics, they too can be star athletes or play professional sports.

All of us who have witnessed youth sports or have had children participate in them can probably recall a handful of athletes who have had absolutely no specialty training—often little coaching—and who just seem to get it. These are the kids who seem to be faster than everybody else, can hit a baseball farther or throw it faster. A kid with very little athletic ability or natural speed will be hard-pressed to become a star athlete, no matter how many coaching clinics or sports performance centers he attends. I'm not saying that we should discourage these youngsters from participating in performance centers or clinics. I do believe that parents and well-meaning coaches sometimes put unrealistic expectations on these types of athletes, which creates undue stress for children who may be better off doing something else.

Perhaps a child like this has natural ability in another area, such as music or the performing arts. Maybe they're a very good student and would rather participate in science and academia. We need to find the natural bent of each child and help to train them accordingly. Although dad may have been a star baseball player or football player, his young son might not have the knack or the desire for it. In my opinion, and based on my professional experience, trying to force a square peg into a round hole only leads to extreme frustration for the child and the parent as well.

You can often hear these parents at youth sporting events, yelling from the stands, "Why can't you do it? Run faster. Tackle him!" All who have witnessed this have felt somewhat embarrassed for the parent and for the poor child who is doing the best they can. A wise coach of mine once said that coaching takes place before and after an athletic event as a parent. During the event, a parent's job is to encourage and to give a simple smile to their child as they participate because, after all, isn't it supposed to be fun?

While I believe that sports performance centers can help certain athletes and certainly serve a vital purpose in instructing athletes on proper form and technique, many people place false hope in these centers as panaceas for every child who wants to become a star athlete. As long as realistic expectations are maintained, these centers can help kids get out of the house and develop courage to participate in sports that they may enjoy but are just lacking in certain areas to become better. Each child is different. Some children are going to be athletes, some are going to be musicians, and some may become doctors and politicians. It's important to remember that when our children participate in sports.

While everybody benefits from participating in sports because of the physical fitness aspect, not everybody will be a star. The sooner we realize and accept this, the better it is for ourselves and our children. Accepting this will lead to less frustration and maybe some money saved from not participating in specialty camps and sports performance centers. That money could be used for a family to take a much-needed vacation and reconnect.

I don't think the parents or the coaches are to blame. With all of the glitz and the glamour shown in the media surrounding professional athletes, there's a natural tendency for every young boy and girl to want to do that, even if that's not their specific area of talent. It's our job as coaches and parents to try to discover our children's natural talents and encourage them in those directions. That is how we will help our children excel and find success.

Friday Night Lights

Several years ago, when I still lived in California, I read a *Time* magazine article about the abuse of steroids in high-school athletes. The article was quite disturbing, as it exposed the number of adolescent athletes using performance-enhancing drugs to try to gain an edge on the competition. The article focused on Texas football in particular, but when I was still in California, I did not appreciate the difference between high-school football in California and high-school football in Texas.

If you've seen the movie *Friday Night Lights*, I don't need to say more. When I first arrived in Texas, driving through Odessa, Texas, which is where the movie *Friday Night Lights* was based on the Permian Panthers, I saw stadiums as big as any college stadium I had seen in California. It quickly became apparent that the emphasis on football and performance was something much different than I had experienced in California. It was not uncommon for children born in local hospitals of towns in which these powerhouse football programs were based to be given football jerseys or cheer outfits before they even left the hospital, when they were still in the nursery. Now that's indoctrination.

With all of this fanfare and pressure to perform, it's easy to see how many of these young, adolescent athletes would want to gain an edge. I remember the peer pressure and the social implications when playing football and other high-school sports. If you're a good athlete, you are often more popular or dating one of the cheerleaders. It's also possible that you'll get out of your small town and have the opportunity to play your sport at the next level, obtaining a college education. Many well-meaning parents see football and athletics as a way out. I think that was certainly the case in the movie *Friday Night Lights* in Odessa, Texas at that time.

The *Time* article went on to explain how one particular, well-known football player in Texas had committed suicide. One of the main side effects of steroids can be major depression and altered body image. People who take steroids never believe they're big enough. They get paranoid and extremely aggressive, and this does not even touch on all of the physical side effects and health risks of steroids.

Many professional athletes in the NFL, when asked if they knew that they could only play their sport for a limited period of time, have fame and fortune, and then die after, would they do it again, many would answer with a resounding, "Yes." I think that answer illustrates how sideways and unbalanced our culture has become, that some of the most important people now—the people that our children hold as role models—are high-paid athletes.

USA Today published an article that claimed Frisco, Texas and North Texas in general as the best place to raise an athlete in the entire United States. There's certainly support for that. When there are so many sports performance programs, there is sports specialization, which leads to the epidemics of injuries that I see.

There is a philosophy that is bred into young children. My youngest boy experienced it when he moved to Texas with us from San Diego, California. He wanted to play soccer, football, and other sports, but his coaches told him that he had to choose. He was nine years old. Some even suggested that he pick a position and focus on that. We didn't have him do that, but as he entered high school, we faced this challenge again; he was told that he would have to choose a sport.

My son had not participated in soccer for several years and was told that he probably wouldn't make the varsity team because he hadn't been playing year-round, which would put him at a disadvantage. As a proud father, I am happy to say that my son did make the varsity team. I really believe that he is an athlete in the sense that he is strong, and he is fast. Those natural abilities carry through multiple sports.

Although he hadn't necessarily been playing soccer for the last several years, nor had he participated in sports specialization, some athletes are naturally talented and able to cross over into many sports, as it says in The Sports Gene book. The skills that are obtained in many sports can cross over and help children to be better athletes while giving their bodies a chance to rest while they're developing. It requires a lot of energy and a lot of calories for a young, skeletally immature body to grow.

When young athletes stress their bodies beyond their ability to repair, that's when breakdown occurs. Stress fractures are one of the most common things that I see. A stress fracture is a clear pathologic condition that indicates a young athlete has done too much, too soon or too often. The body breaks down and doesn't have the opportunity or enough time to heal itself. Many parents come into my office concerned about a potential injury and say, "We certainly want to find out what's wrong with our child and do whatever is best for them, Doctor."

I always appreciate hearing that, but far too often that statement is followed with, "When can they get back on the field? When can they play again? When will they be ready? They're ten years old, Doctor, but they have a really important showcase coming up next weekend."

Or they say, "Doctor, my 11-year-old is participating in a gymnastics competition at Nationals. It's very important."

When I, as a father or as a physician, look the parents in the eye and tell them that the child needs to rest, you would think I had just given them a death sentence and told them that there was no hope left. One of the biggest roles that I play in North Texas as a sports medicine specialist is having serious conversations with parents and helping reset their expectations for what is important for their children.

I jokingly question the young athletes in the presence of their parents: "How much are you getting paid to play baseball? How much are you getting paid to compete in gymnastics? How much are you getting paid to be on that soccer team?"

They'll usually laugh it off and say, "Well, it's nothing, but maybe someday, Doc!" Even in the joke there's some truth. There is the hope of getting a scholarship and money; maybe fame, maybe fortune.

Unfortunately, in my experience, you either have it, or you don't. Drew Brees, one of the most famous and recognized quarterbacks, never even started playing football until he was a freshman. Other athletes didn't start participating until later in life. Those are the athletes I use as references: If you really want to be great, and you really want to succeed, look at what many of the great ones did. When they were nine and ten years old, they were at the sandlot. They were playing with their buddies on the street corner until the streetlights came on. They weren't playing football year-round.

One of the scariest things that's come to North Texas is year-round tackle football for pee wee and youth. It's especially scary given the recently released movie Concussion and the focus on concussion and head-injury prevention. As a husband, a father, and a sports medicine specialist, I think that year-round tackle football for pee wee and youth is atrocious.

LaDainian Tomlinson was our running back in San Diego when I was there. He was #5 when playing at TCU, and he set all sorts of records. He was one of the most exciting running backs I ever had a chance to work with, and he was an even better man. I remember many conversations with LaDainian about one of his mentors and heroes: the famous Cowboy, Emmitt Smith.

LaDainian said that when he was a young man, he was fortunate enough to go to a football camp that was put on by Emmitt Smith. It was at that football camp that LaDainian knew what he wanted to do. He wanted to play football. Some of the most important advice that LaDainian Tomlinson got from Emmitt Smith applies today and should apply to every parent who wants their son to play football and be great. Emmitt Smith told LaDainian that you only have so many hits in your career: Know when to put your head down; know when to step out of bounds. That's certainly sound advice given to an elite running back. A young athlete and their parents should meditate on that.

Many fans and others in the U.S. are probably aware of Junior Seau taking his own life in San Diego. I had the privilege of knowing and working with Junior Seau. He was probably one of the most outstanding linebackers to ever play the game. He was in the Hall of Fame. As the movie *Concussion* showed, we now have a better understanding of head injuries and the dangers of them. Although we shouldn't completely speculate on what led to the tragic end of a great man like Junior Seau, all of us parents, coaches, and athletic trainers need to step back and think about whether we really need our kids taking so many shots to the head early on. If we are going to play sports, we need to be smart about it.

I love what my boys learned on the football field, and I would still choose to have them play football. They learned about leadership. They learned that it's not about me, but about the team. They learned if you want to achieve more, you need to do more. They learned on the football field that you better show up early because being on time is late. You better know your job, and you better do your job. When practice is over, don't be the first to leave; ask if there's more that you can do. If you want to play on Friday night, you better practice during the week.

The old phrase coaches would say is, "Practice like you play." I'm not sure that means that in practice you need to try to take off your teammate's head or 'ear hole' them, which means tackling with helmet-to-helmet. This can lead to young kids developing concussions before they've even had the opportunity to play at a level that matters, like in college or professionally.

My youngest boy, who played high-school football and plays intramural football at Baylor University, told me that during almost every game his ears ring. That probably means that in just about every game my son is having a minor concussion.

We parents and coaches need to step back and say, "Should we be doing more?" For all of the glory of Friday nights, I have often lectured parents and families not to be surprised if football goes away in North Texas and in the

United States. Coaches and parents look at me and say, "Are you crazy? Football is never going away."

Roger Goodell, the commissioner of the NFL, understood that the NFL needed to own head injuries, so they formed their own group to focus on them. That's what we need to do at the youth level to prevent head injuries. Because of the devastating concussions, head injuries, and deaths that have occurred in North Texas to football players, football programs will no longer be able to obtain insurance. When that happens, football programs will cease to exist. With no money, there's no mission, and there's no football.

Psych Issues: Anxiety and Depression

Depression and suicide among athletes is a real problem. We place so much pressure on young, immature children to perform or risk having no value beyond a sport. We place pressure on them that if they don't get scholarships, they can't go to college. This leads to the use of performance-enhancing drugs (PEDs). The side effects of PEDs are associated depression and anxiety. Young athletes use alcohol to "steady their nerves" and treat the anxiety that's created by feeling inadequate.

There are some primary and secondary issues associated with anxiety and depression. Parents and coaches place such pressure on kids to perform for the false hope of acquiring scholarships that it can lead to minor and/or major depression and/or anxiety issues in young athletes. The extreme pressure that kids feel between trying to balance sports and school is very challenging. Often athletes feel like they're letting down their parents or their coaches. They feel stressed or anxious because of the demands of school. Most schools have gotten rid of recess at the elementary level and physical education as well. Kids spend more time in classrooms and are given more homework. Then they come home and have to go to practices and games.

Weekends are often spent away at events and tournaments.

At a young age they feel that there's just not enough time to get things done. Adults are able to cope and to deal with those stresses more readily because our brains are fully developed. Children's brains are not fully developed, so they're not able to process that stress as well, and it certainly leads to depression and anxiety. I think it can also lead to a condition called somatization, which causes children to experience physical symptoms as a result of the stress and anxiety they feel because there's just so much to do in a day.

One of the secondary causes of depression and anxiety in athletes, one that's not often talked about, is the use of performance-enhancing drugs at very young ages. More and more young athletes use performance-enhancing drugs. One legal performance-enhancing drug is caffeine. How many kids in elementary school, as well as in junior high and high school, use coffee and even energy drinks such as Monster Energy and Red Bull daily. Caffeine can certainly cause anxiety, a rapid heartbeat, and tachycardia, which can give a child a sense of anxiety.

Other lesser known substances that are used include anabolic steroids and growth hormones.

Anabolic steroids can cause depression, as well as anger and roid rage personality disorders.

There is increasing pressure on young athletes to perform at very high levels in order to obtain scholarships. That false hope of obtaining scholarships drives athletes to make decisions that they may not otherwise make. The use of performance-enhancing drugs certainly can be a risk factor for those types of psychological issues.

Regulating Sports

I am the last person in the world who would usually advocate for more regulations of anything; however, when children are at stake, everything changes. As a parent and a physician, I feel a strong need to have some guidelines and regulations to protect our children. When I see a ten-year-old pitcher who has destroyed his elbow and needs to have surgery, that is inexcusable. These types of injuries are completely preventable. If someone had adhered to guidelines about pitch counts or simply listened to the child when they started to complain that their elbow hurt, that child would not be "retiring" at ten years old.

Too often coaches or parents have their own agendas. I am sure no one ever thinks that their actions will cause harm, but they don't really understand the danger of not resting young athletes and limiting their training or competition. Young bodies are growing and developing, and they need rest. Unfortunately, many young athletes play on two or three baseball teams, are involved in offseason performance/conditioning, and meet with pitching and hitting coaches several times per week. Then parents wonder why their children's bodies get hurt.

In high school there is "voluntary" off-season training. The truth is that most off-season training is far from voluntary because everyone knows who attends. Players are played against each other, and coaches penalize those who don't show up. Athletes are often injured in the season, go straight into off-season, then pre-season, and back into the regular season without ever having the chance to heal from their injuries.

It is very sad when you see grown men treat boys with such little care or concern. These coaches really do believe that beating kids down makes them stronger. I couldn't disagree more. There is a point at which you can break someone's spirit. When someone is really injured, and you make fun of them and degrade them in front of their friends, it causes resentment and discourages them. Very few athletes turn this criticism into motivation, which is what the coaches intend.

Great coaches know that you must lead some athletes differently. Some respond to strong words and discipline, while others fold if handled this way. Most athletes need encouragement to excel, and many young men do not have solid role models. They do not have fathers around, or the fathers they do have don't help them to feel loved and nurtured. It is a great lie that men must be yelled at or "broken" to become strong. This is why I believe we have so many dysfunctional families and men; no one has set the example. Young boys get treated harshly by grown men and then repeat the cycle with their own children. Many young boys have inner anger, but most just want to know that a man in their life really loves them and wants them to succeed. The dangerous cycle repeats itself until someone has the courage to say, "No more." It is no wonder that so many coaches seem angry and treat their athletes in the same way they were treated. Sports should teach young men about teamwork and hard work. Sports should not be about breaking young men down and discouraging them. Unfortunately, one broken man can't lead another effectively.

Tony Dungy, former coach of the Indianapolis Colts, knows how to coach winners. In Tony's book Uncommon he talks about his football coach at the University of Minnesota. Tony remembers his coach telling the players that common men were just that: common. His coach was looking for uncommon men. Tony goes on to say that this was a turning point for him. He realized that as a young player he must be set apart. If he wanted to be great, he couldn't be like the other guys. Is it any wonder that Tony became not only a talented football player with the Pittsburgh Steelers but arguably one of the greatest coaches of all time?

Tony understood how men need to be led and that many are broken themselves. When an athlete knows you truly love them and care about them, they will perform for you. As parents and coaches, getting the best out of children should be what we are after.

Considering that many coaches won't look out for their athletes, we as physicians and parents must. With coaches pushing "voluntary practices" and violating league rules, someone has to have their back. I believe there needs to be rules in place and enforced that prevent players from meeting "voluntarily" before pre-season. Athletes should not be forced to participate in other activities that they do not want to participate in, just because a coach thinks it will make them better. If during pre-season an athlete is not good enough or is unprepared, the situation will sort itself out. Athletes should not have to wake up at 5 AM and lift weights before school, so they can be tired all day and fall asleep in class, only to then be required to go to a "volunteer" after-school practice. We wonder why we have an epidemic problem of young men with ADD, who can't focus in the classroom. They are tired. Young men need rest so their bodies can grow.

How do I know this works on a practical level? My son played football for a local high school that lost every single game, except one, over a three-year period. As the team performed worse and worse, the coaches blamed the athletes even though these same athletes won many games together in junior high.

At this school there was no off-season for football. The boys were "punished" for losing by being forced to work out harder and longer, and more "voluntary" off-season practice was required. If you were injured, you were openly made fun of or told that you were "faking it" in front of your peers.

A friend of my son's broke his wrist in a game, and despite X-rays and a doctor's note, his coaches made fun of him, calling him "soft" and "weak." This young man went on to play with a cast, despite having a broken wrist, because he felt pressure and humiliation from his coaches. Unfortunately, the trauma from playing and getting tackled caused the fracture not to heal, and he needed to have surgery. Even after undergoing surgery, his coaches wanted him to lift, and he was made fun of for not being able to do so. His spirit and his body broken, he never played football again.

At another high school in the same town as the school above, the practices were shorter, there was very little mandatory lifting, and the young men were encouraged and loved. There was no cursing and no making fun of an athlete in front of his peers. If you were hurt, you took time to heal. There were no "volunteer" workouts or requirements to do multiple sports and lift weights before school. While the other football team in the same town could barely win one game in three years, this high school went undefeated in league play and made it to the state finals in Texas two years in a row.

In medicine we would call this a controlled study. As a parent, what team do you want your kid to play for? Do you want your child to be encouraged, loved, and taught perseverance, or broken down, discouraged, and have their spirit broken?

The year before my son's team went to the state finals, they did not make playoffs. For the three years prior, they had a coach like the other school, who overworked the athletes and broke their spirits. This coach was fired. Next year, with the same athletes, the team went undefeated in the district and went to the Texas TAPPS State Finals in football.

Was this a coincidence? Maybe, but I think the other coach knew how to coach young men. Instead of breaking men down, he built them up. As the football team got further along in its season, practices got shorter, and there was very little weightlifting at all. This coach understood that the game itself breaks down athletes' bodies, and he wanted his boys healthy to win games. His ego was not tied up in whether he could break these young men down. Instead, he built them up. I would even say that the other high school had far more talent and resources than my son's high school. The difference was in the coaching!

It breaks my heart to see young men's spirits broken and great athletes ruined by coaches who are broken themselves. I don't think it is often as much of a head problem as it is a heart problem. As a physician, I have taken care of coaches and many young men. I realize there is tremendous pressure on coaches to succeed, or risk losing their jobs. I am not willing, however, to sacrifice my child to coaches' egos. We need to start training coaches and mentoring them. We need more men like Tony Dungy, who teach coaches to train athletes in a way that gets the best out of them.

One thing I can't understand is how coaches who break young men down and fail to win a single game are allowed to keep their jobs. Even crazier is how parents keep giving their children to these coaches. All of us must hold coaches and parents accountable if we are to protect are children's spirits and bodies. Very few athletes will play sports after high school, but their bodies must last a lifetime. Tell an athlete or any child for long enough that he is a loser or a failure, and he will prove you right. Let all of us who are involved with athletes strive to be encouragers and use training techniques that create winners. Just because coaches have done it that way for a hundred years doesn't make it right. Just like Tony Dungy said, "Don't be common; be uncommon."

Select Snobs

Anybody who's been in youth sports for any time at all has come across a group of parents that are "select snobs." Within the first five minutes of talking to them, these parents tell you about how Susie or Johnny plays on an expensive select team. Usually, they recount for the listener how much money it costs to be on the team, the extreme tryouts that their child had to go through to make the team, and all the exotic travel that they must endure to be on the select team.

Young children are flown around the United States and other parts of the world to play in select tournaments. I've seen this phenomenon happen as young as seven and eight years of age. Such teams also tend to be year-round and require high levels of commitment from families, as well as the children.

Often families have to put their own personal lives and jobs on hold in order to take their children on these long trips, often causing the child to miss school. Some of these young children and their families even have private tutors that travel with them, so being on the move doesn't affect their studies. While I know that for gymnasts and ice skaters this is more commonplace, I also see it happen for select soccer, hockey, lacrosse, and golf players as well.

While kids may enjoy doing whatever sport it is that they do, I believe that once they get to this level of select, parents need to step back and ask themselves, "Who am I doing this for? Am I doing this for my child, or am I doing this for my own ego?" Sometimes a group of these parents get together, and it seems like a contest of who can one-up the other ones in terms of whose select team is more expensive, who travels more, and who spends more.

From my own personal observation, it seems that a lot of these "select athletes" are not what I would classify as gifted or exemplary. Even though you can't buy talent, it seems at times that parents try to buy slot on high-school teams in hopes of future scholarships.

It has become commonplace for high schools to begin scouting for kids for their teams as young as eight or nine years old, and the process has become very political. If a child hasn't participated in a select team, they may not have a chance to make a high-school team because coaches perceive them as not being serious. This has created such an imbalance in the lives of young children that many have, in my opinion, lost their youth.

A young patient of mine, who is an outstanding baseball player and had focused much of his time on developing those skills, decided he wanted to play football for a local high school. The patient had played when he was a sophomore and was quite good but did not play his junior year and was unable to play spring football going into his senior year because of baseball commitments and because he was shunned by the high-school coaching staff.

The coaches told him that he could not play football his senior year because he had not played his junior year and because he had not played spring football. They would not even give this young athlete a chance to compete for a position on the team. It is unfortunate that pride would stand in the way of a team acquiring a great athlete that could positively contribute.

Unfortunately, this young athlete was not originally from this particular geographic area; he had moved in late to school, so he was not well known to the coaches. This young athlete did not have a dad who was a coach on the football team or contributed a lot of money to the booster club, so he was simply looked over.

The last I knew of this young athlete, his family was attempting to appeal to the athletic director and the school board to allow him even the chance to try out and participate on his high-school team.

How unfortunate that a young, high-school athlete, who was simply participating in another sport, couldn't even try out, let alone play, for his own high-school team as a senior. I'm sure that if he does not get to play, this will be a memory that he will carry the rest of his life. It's an example of coaches at the high-school level perpetuating the select snob phenomenon.

When do well-meaning parents become snobs? When sports become more about the parent and less about the young athlete. If you, as a parent, find yourself at the country club or at a cocktail party spending more time talking about what it costs to participate on the select team, who is on your select team, or how many frequent-flyer miles you earn by traveling for the select team, you can classify yourself as a select snob.

During the time that I wrote this book, several friends had children who could not go on family vacations, could not have sleepovers with their friends, could not take daytrips to the lake, and could not simply be kids because they spent the summer traveling the United States for either select baseball or select soccer teams.

If you were to talk to any of these kids one-on-one, they would tell you that all they want to do is stay home and hang out with their friends. It's fine for a parent to encourage their child and help them to be disciplined and committed to a team, but parents have to be careful about making sure that they're thinking more about their children than about themselves.

What if they say they're only doing it to give their child a chance, so their child can get a scholarship, so their child can get an education at a good school? Those would be noble motivations for participating in select teams and private-coaching clinics if the statistics backed them up.

Unfortunately, an article on June 27, 2008 in *Smart Money* by Anne Kadet, showed that only 2% of high-school athletes will ever receive a scholarship and that the average award, if given, is usually less than $10,000. This is often less than the cost of what private lessons, select teams, and equipment costs.

The larger cost is the time that can never be regained from participating in all of those year-round select sports and private lessons. Many kids will grow up to resent having lost time that they will never get back again. I'm not sure that you can put a price tag on what that costs.

When considering whether or not to put your child on one of these select teams and considering the low percentage of those who earn scholarships, consider the cost of college. If you really were doing something just for the sake of your child getting a scholarship to pay for a good education, would you have been better off investing your money to pay for your child's education?

A study completed by *The New York Times* and published in March 2008 revealed some disturbing facts for parents hoping for scholarships. NCAA athletic scholarships rarely are full rides. They average out to $8,707, according to this study. In sports like track-and-field and baseball, the number is only $2,000. If you average the amount for football, it rises to roughly $10,409. Tuition and room-and-board at an NCAA institution often costs between $20,000 and $50,000 a year.

In a recent 2003-2004 study, the best-paying sport for scholarship at the NCAA level is, surprisingly, neither football nor men's or women's basketball. It's ice hockey, with scholarships at approximately $21,755 a year for men and with women at $20,540. Baseball was the second-lowest men's sport in terms of scholarship, with an average of $5,806.

If these numbers don't support putting children in sports for the scholarship money, and more could be made for children's education by putting money into a college tax-deferred fund, then why do parents continue to throw thousands of dollars at select sports and private coaches every year?

I'm sure there is more than one parent who believes that their child will be that one-in-a-million athlete who beats the odds. Unfortunately, many parents put their children in sports for the wrong reasons, including reliving the glory that they once achieved themselves or living out the glory through their children that they never achieved themselves.

Select sports may afford a child greater exposure to scouts and potential for scholarships and advancement in their athletic event, but the odds are against them. As long as parents and athletes understand and accept the odds and the costs, financially and emotionally, then it may be okay for that particular athlete and family.

If, however, it causes a single mom to have to work multiple jobs and sacrifice time with her children, then my personal opinion is that the money would be best invested in a tax-deferred college fund, and her time would be better invested in spending it with her children because she will never get that back.

It is getting harder and harder for parents to resist the temptation of the world and society that we live in, but if we are to preserve our own sanity and the safety and well-being of our children, then enough is enough; we need to put our money where our mouths are and do the right thing for our children.

Choosing to Play Just One Sport

Nike understood it well and coined the term "cross-training". What happened? In the sports medicine world, we call athletes choosing to play just one sport sports specialization, and it's a bad decision. The reason it happens is the hope of obtaining a scholarship. By sports specializing at a very young age, a child doesn't get the opportunity to rest. Young bodies, muscles, and joints do not have the time to recover. If a child plays on a baseball team, either at school or for a select team, on six, sometimes seven, days a week, that means they are throwing a baseball and hitting a ball without giving their joints the opportunity to ever fully recover. Being skeletally immature means that a child is not done growing, and their young bodies are more prone to injury. Add in lack of sleep because of the increased demands in school, and they are set up for failure.

Encouraging a wide variety of sports, like Nike did back in the '80s during the "Bo Knows" marketing campaign is a healthier way to think about sports. When I grew up, we went from playing football to playing soccer to running track. All of those different sports can actually help you to be a better athlete in the other sports you play; you become more well-rounded. If you play one sport year-round, your body never has a chance to recover.

An interesting study was done a few years ago that looked at baseball players, specifically pitchers, who had longevity, and their risk of injury. The higher rate of injuries among baseball players and specifically pitchers occurred in warm climates. If the player played in a cooler or more northern climate, such as Illinois, Michigan, Minnesota, or Maine, they were less likely to have an injury.

Why? Weather actually forces you to rest in climates where there is snow or other inclement weather. When you live in a warmer climate, where there are more days of sun, you have a higher rate of injury because you are able to participate more often and year-round.

We need to make sure that athletes have the opportunity to develop their musculoskeletal system and not overuse them. Jim Andrews, a very famous and well-known sports-medicine specialist and now the founder of the Andrews Institute, is a very big proponent of athletes participating in multiple sports and is an opponent of sports specialization because of what I've mentioned.

Athletes who participate in one sport at younger ages are at significantly higher risk of enduring career-ending injuries. I see baseball players at nine and ten years of age who have career-ending elbow injuries because they have been playing year-round baseball since they were six or seven years old, pitching multiple times a week, and not adhering to any kind of pitch count.

A pitch count is something that every parent or coach who has a skeletally immature pitcher should consider. There are limits on the number of pitches that a young pitcher should throw each week. These aren't often adhered to because if you are a great pitcher at a very young age, then every coach wants you on their team. Those coaches want to win, and so do your fellow players, so they encourage you to pitch every game. When it's in the bottom of the ninth inning, and you already hit your pitch count, but you're only one or two strikes away from winning the game, a coach is in a very awkward and challenging situation. Do they do the right thing and pull someone off the mound, protecting that child, or do they win the game? That's something that all coaches, parents, and athletes need to be very aware of.

The Sandlot: Where Did It Go?

The Sandlot and the reference to it comes from a very famous movie: *The Sandlot.* Before the advent of cellphones, when you came home from school at the end of the day, you usually got together with your buddies at the cul-de-sac or the end of the street, picked teams, and maybe played baseball. The instructions from moms were, "Be home by the time the streetlights come on for dinner and to get your homework done." You would play sport for the love of sport.

The Sandlot refers to that local community area, maybe a sandlot or a field of sand, where athletes would gather friends and participate in all sorts of sports. I feel that that's been lost in America. We've taken physical education out of most schools. Kids have reached epidemic levels of ADD diagnosis and are on medication because we don't let them participate in general recreation, and instead we have an increase in organized, formal sports participation. For all of the anxiety and stress that kids feel, whatever happened to going out and playing with your buddies just because sports are fun?

We've taken the fun out of sports for many kids. A friend of mine is an orthopedic surgeon sports medicine specialist. He takes care of U.S. Olympic gymnasts, and he often tells me that he has seen an increase in injuries, but often these injuries are feigned or faked because the athletes finally reach high school, and they don't want to do the sport anymore. It's lost its fun. It's become a job. It's a means to an end for a scholarship, but the fun is gone.

What happened to the sandlot in society? What happened to participating in sport just for the love of sport?

"Show Me the Money!"

The movie *Jerry Maguire* inspired a generation and highlighted the big money to be made in sports. Having spent a career taking care of professional athletes that get paid millions of dollars, I see firsthand how most young athletes start off, viewing these professionals as their heroes. They want to be them someday. They then ask themselves how they can get there. Often the answer is driven by money rather than love of the sport.

The U.S. Olympics are supposed to represent participation in sports for the love of sports, all the way back to the ancient Greek games, but, of course, sports are entertaining, and with all forms of entertainment comes money. When there's money involved, it certainly drives behavior. At very young ages, kids are drawn to the images they see on TV. That really is what was highlighted in the movie *Jerry Maguire*, where that famous quote, "Show me the money!" originated.

Unfortunately, it's a false premise, and that's why I call it "The Scholarship Myth". To think that if you participate in sports you have a high chance of obtaining a scholarship is false. So is receiving the money in the form of a scholarship and even less likely of ever being able to play a professional sport and being able to be paid for that. Less than 1% to 2% of high-school athletes ever obtain sports scholarships. Of those, it is unlikely that they make it to the professional level.

When most people think of a scholarship, they think of a full-ride scholarship. They don't understand that the vast majority of athletic scholarships, even if you are lucky enough to be among the 1% to 2% that obtain them, are year-to-year scholarships. Coaches can pull those scholarships for other athletes or divert those monies to other programs or other athletes at their discretion.

If you went to a very expensive school that you could not have otherwise afforded, and you get injured, you're now in the very difficult predicament of not being able to participate in athletics. If you're only able to be at that school because of the sports scholarship that you have lost, you may have to leave that school and not complete your education. This puts families and athletes in very compromised positions.

The bottom line is that the money is not what people think. As a parent, you would be wiser to take those dollars and invest them in funds for education, saving for college instead of investing them in coaching, sports specialization and training, and after-school sports-performance programs, which are very prominent now. I think that most people and most parents don't want to admit that you have to win a little bit of the genetic race if you want to be successful in sports.

If your parents were short, it is very unlikely that you can do anything you want if you just put your mind to it, despite what your mama told you. You're probably not going to grow up and be an NBA center. On the other hand, we know from a very good book called *The Sports Gene* that we can identify genetic factors that predispose someone to success in a certain sport. You have to win a little bit of the genetic race to be successful, and even then the odds are stacked against you when it comes to obtaining money for scholarships and being paid to play a professional sport.

Although I played sports at all levels, and my kids played sports in high school and into college, and although I think it is healthy for kids to participate in sports, we should have balance and emphasize education above sports. Most people know that the acronym NFL stands for "National Football League." If you are fortunate enough to make it there, a little joke is that NFL stands for "not for long."

Even if you make it into the NFL, the average NFL career is about three years. In dealing with NFL athletes who are finally fortunate enough to make it to that level, I have seen them squander those dollars and become penniless and bankrupt in years after entering their professional careers.

JaMarcus Russell was signed with the Los Angeles Raiders, and I believe had a guaranteed $45 million. Unfortunately, something happened to him that happens to many young athletes who were very successful in college: He went into the NFL, squandered his dollars, and was penniless and broke in a matter of years.

As parents, it is important that we have our children participate in sports because they're fun, they're healthy, and they burn off stress and anxiety, helping children to focus on their education. Really we should put education first. Sports have their role, but they probably shouldn't be the primary focus for most kids. "Show me the money!" should not be the emphasis. It should be, "Show me the grades!" or, "Show me the focus on education!" That's what will help most children and most young people have the most success.

Coaches and Training Techniques

You need to ask yourself, "Who's on my team?" An athlete always needs to know who is on their team. Likewise, parents need to know who is on their kid's teams. Who is the athletic trainer taking care of their athletes?

Take football, for example. Who is on the sidelines on Friday nights? Is the athletic trainer at all of the practices? Knowing who is on the team and when they show up is important. Knowing the coach, knowing what their philosophy is, and knowing whether they are someone who thinks that restricting water from athletes is a punishment or if athletes should get water regularly so they can perform well is important.

You should know who your team physician is. Is he a sports medicine specialist? Is he just somebody who was available to stand on the sidelines?

It's important for every parent at the beginning of every football season to know who will be taking care of their children. If I really wanted my kid to play a particular sport, I wouldn't hesitate to change coaches or teams if I didn't feel like those coaches were in line with my philosophy and put my kid's health before winning.

Heat and Hydration

Having relocated from California to Texas, I've had to deal with an extreme change in climate. Southern California, where I grew up and played most of my sports, is a very mild climate. When temperatures did get into the triple digits, we did not deal with humidity. Coaches and physicians certainly can't control the climate, but it's something that they can be aware of and monitor to prevent heat illness in athletes.

In the area of Texas where I live, it is common to see triple digits throughout the late summer. This is about the time football teams start their two-a-day practices. These can be a prescription for disaster. Every year several high-school athletes lose their lives from complications related to heat illness. The sad thing about heat-related deaths is that they are preventable.

An athlete who becomes overheated and is left to himself will seek to cool himself by removing clothing, seeking shade, drinking water, and removing himself from whatever event he is participating in. It is only when athletes feel pressure from coaches or other individuals that they avoid protecting themselves from excessive heat. This is vitally important for coaches, parents, and athletes to understand.

The trouble that I see as a physician is when coaches with the old-school mentality use water breaks or a lack thereof as rewards or punishments for athletes who are or are not working hard. When my son first started playing high-school football, coaches would tell the players that they would not get water unless they worked harder, or they were required to run more plays before being "rewarded" with water breaks.

This is very dangerous behavior for those who are in positions to protect our children. It is this philosophy that leads to needless deaths every year. Many coaches will also not allow particular football players to remove their helmets during practice, which further complicates the problem.

More than 70% of a person's heat is dissipated from their head and neck region. In order for an athlete to be able to cool himself, he must be able to expose the head and neck region to the environment for heat radiation or evaporation.

When you are faced with high humidity, which is not uncommon for areas of Texas and other parts of the United States, sweat sits on the body and does not evaporate, which makes it even more difficult for an athlete to cool.

I've heard many coaches say that they let kids drink when they are thirsty. This philosophy is also problematic because thirst has been shown in numerous studies to be a poor indicator of hydration. In fact, literature supports that when thirst is used as an indicator for hydration, you will be approximately 50% behind on fluid balance.

Instead, water and fluids that are cool should be readily available to athletes, and coaches should make it a requirement during training to drink and rehydrate. This should be encouraged and mandated by coaches and should not be used as a reward or punishment for athletes.

In fact, for every hour of practice, athletes should stop halfway through that hour and hydrate with at least eight ounces of cool water. It is not uncommon for an athlete to lose more than a liter of sweat per hour of exercise, and they can lose up to two liters per hour of exercise. Sweating is a very effective manner of cooling the body, but it can lead to significant fluid loss if the water is not replenished.

One good way to monitor fluid loss is with weight. Weighing athletes before and after practice and looking for a change in body weight can indicate a hydration problem. An athlete who has sustained fluid loss over a long period of time is at significant risk for heat intolerance.

A loss of greater than 2% to 3% of body fluid from sweating causes an increase in core temperature that is proportional to the amount of dehydration. If an athlete loses greater than 5% of their body weight, there is a marked risk in heat intolerance. Athletes who lose more than 7% of their body weight due to sweat loss are susceptible to fatal heatstroke from the cumulative effects of hypohydration.

This becomes increasingly important when athletes participate in successive daily exercise activities or even two-a-days in football programs. Athletes with body weight losses of more than 2% to 3% per practice should be reminded to drink extra fluids and can compete within 1 to 2 pounds of their starting weights from the previous day.

An athlete who has losses of 5% to 6% is already at a mildly severe deficit. These athletes should be restricted to participating in only light workouts after hydrating to their normal weights. Athletes with more than 7% loss of body weight represent severe water depletion and should not participate in sports but instead be examined by a physician.

An important thing for coaches to have, especially in areas where it's hot and humid, is a wet bulb. Standard temperatures give inadequate information for coaches to decide whether it is safe to practice. A wet bulb globe temperature index is the most commonly used indicator by athletic trainers and physicians to decide when it is safe to practice and at what level.

The use of the wet bulb is especially important when individuals exercise in humid areas. When an area has humidity of 60% or greater, sweat is not evaporated unless there is air movement. You can see how training in a very hot, humid climate with no breeze could cause an athlete to be at risk for heat illness, especially when you consider that evaporation represents somewhere between 70% and 80% of heat loss. If a football player, for example, is wearing a helmet and shoulder pads, with their neck and head covered, and it is hot and humid, they're going to be in trouble unless the coach takes specific action to prevent heat illness.

Some coaches will say that they consult the weather service and use general temperature, humidity, and wind speed as broad guidelines. These are often highly inaccurate for specific exercise locations. A wet bulb temperature index should be taken on the athletic field where the athletes practice in order to properly assess the situation.

This is also vitally important for athletes who practice on artificial turf fields, where the temperature can be much greater than it would be on a grass field. Using general weather reports would not take into account these unique circumstances.

Clothing is very important for keeping athletes cool as well. Recently, many clothing manufacturers have developed new fabrics that allow athletes to have improved cooling. Small holes in fabric that is light and breathes improves evaporation and cooling as well.

Many parents ask about replacement drinks, such as Gatorade®, POWERADE®, etc. In general, these do not offer any greater benefits over the short-term; however, for athletes participating in extremely long practices, especially back-to-back practices like two-a-days in football or consecutive days of practice in extreme heat and humidity, carbohydrate-loaded drinks help to hydrate and restore some of the glucose stores that may be lost.

Another common recommendation that I make is to avoid caffeinated beverages, as caffeine may have a negative effect on athletic performance in heat. Small doses of caffeine have not been shown to be a diuretic, which some people have inaccurately reported before, but they can adversely affect the autonomic and nervous system, inhibiting normal cooling mechanisms.

One of the signs that parents and coaches can look for is heat cramps. These are painful contractions that usually affect large muscle groups, such as the thigh and sometimes the buttocks. Heat cramps often start in one area and travel to another. Treatment for muscle cramps include stretching and fluid and electrolyte replacement. When severe, they sometimes require IV fluids.

Heat illness is something that parents and coaches must understand is not a single point but is a timeline or a continuum that starts with heat syncope or heat cramps and progresses to heatstroke, which can be fatal in 50% to 70% of cases. It is this level of heat illness that leads to the several deaths of high-school athletes every year.

Being aware of heat illness is vitally important for parents, coaches, and athletes. Having planned strategies for hydrating athletes in hot and humid climates is vitally important for keeping athletes safe. Adequately hydrated athletes have been shown to perform better and to have lower incidences of injuries. Cool water readily available to athletes is usually adequate, and glucose-supplemented flavored drinks can be used for intense training or athletes participating in vigorous consecutive days of training.

If athletes are suspected of having heat illness, they should be removed from the athletic event, and cooling measures should be started. If severe, medical treatment should be urgently sought. I recommend a wet bulb for all high-school athletic programs and using a standard chart to assess the risk of heat illness.

Heat illness is a very real concern for athletes participating in hot and humid climates; however, if adequate precautions are taken, the risk can be greatly reduced. Preventing catastrophic consequences requires communication between athletes, coaches, and often parents. The old adage of "You can lead a horse to water, but you can't make him drink" does not apply to athletes. In this case, you need to lead the athlete to the water, have it readily available, and ensure that they drink it.

When Did Cheerleading Become Competitive Gymnastics?

When I played football and sports, the stereotypical cheerleader was the popular girl who went all out is what we would call as cheer. They would be out on Friday nights, shouting cheers, leading the crowd in cheers, and encouraging the athletes on the field. Somewhere along the way, cheerleaders no longer stood on their boxes with their bullhorns, shouting out cheers, but became gymnasts.

In order to actually make a high-school cheerleading squad in the state of Texas, you better be able to do round-off back handsprings and have spent some time with world-famous WOGA (World Olympic Gymnastics Academy). It's now become a requirement for cheerleaders to be able to tumble, which is a skill that is learned in gymnastics. No longer is it necessarily the 'cool kids' who become the cheerleaders.

Cheerleading is a dangerous sport. Football, rugby, and lacrosse have their injuries, but I see and have taken care of a significant number of cheerleaders with significant injuries, even spine injuries.

When I was at Rancho Los Amigos, USC's rehabilitation hospital in Los Angeles, California, I took care of a cheerleader who was from the

University of Nebraska and who was a flier. That means she was thrown up into the air and caught. Unfortunately, this young lady was not caught and landed on her neck. She became a tetraplegic, or what the lay public would call a "quadriplegic," unable to use her arms or legs. She was vent-dependent for the rest of her life.

It is certainly exciting to watch all of those athletes flying through the air, but it's dangerous. It has become a competition. These young girls and boys often participate in gymnastics in order to gain the skills to make their cheer squads and then will participate in competitive cheerleading teams when they are not obligated to their school activities. It has become a competitive sport and a very lucrative one, in which people, again, pay lots of money to participate.

Cheerleading has also been glorified in movies, including the famous cheerleading movie *Bring It On*, which highlighted competitive cheerleading. Cheerleading has also become a sport that results in a great deal of injuries. Parents, coaches, and athletic trainers should be aware of that and should certainly consider limiting some activities because there is the potential for serious repercussions, including spinal injuries, in particular.

Self-Confidence vs. Self-Esteem

Sometimes the terms "self-confidence" and "self-esteem" are used interchangeably; however, I think that people who sometimes don't feel good about themselves but find themselves successful in a particular sport begin to feel good about themselves. They then have self-confidence, which helps to bring about better self-esteem or a better vision of themselves. Many young kids can certainly gain better feelings about themselves by participating in sports and finding sports that they succeed in. For many young children who may have problems at home, their sports teams become their families.

I was raised by my grandparents and actually spent some time in foster care. One of the ways that I was able to be accepted and to survive in foster care, moving from home to home, was to be fairly good at sports and by getting picked to be on the good teams. Sports probably helped to protect me and to maintain my self-esteem because I had self-confidence in sports.

For people like myself who have gone through those types of things, sports can help them to face challenges, to adapt, and to be accepted by their peers. Right or wrong, still today I think that they're still certainly acceptance of sports and if you're good at a certain sport. Sports can sometimes help to bridge social and social-economic gaps.

Sometimes individuals who come from very different backgrounds find themselves as one on the athletic field. I think this represents one of the greatest parts of America, and seeing people of all colors, all races, and all religions playing sports it certainly helps to build bonds. Wouldn't it be great if all Americans could live like so many people have to live on the fields of athletics in order to win? How much better could we do as a nation if we acted the way that many of our children do on the fields of play?

Sports certainly can help a person to build self-confidence and self-esteem. They can even have an impact on their family and their community as a whole, in addition to their team. I think that many athletes can become great leaders and can certainly impact people in positive ways.

Are Kids Really Better Today?

There's a movie called *Race* that highlights the story of Jesse Owens, going back to the Olympic games when Adolf Hitler presided over them. During those times, athletes had spikes driven into leather-soled shoes that they had to slip on, and they ran on cinder tracks. Now we have special artificial tracks and special shoes. The world records for the 100 meters, the 200 meters, and the 400 meters have certainly been broken, but I think all of us would agree that we're not that much faster.

Football players today are certainly bigger, stronger, and faster, but I'm not sure if that translates into healthier, happier athletes, especially when you consider that because these athletes have gotten bigger, stronger, and faster, their collisions are bigger and harder. That translates into a higher rate of concussion. There are certainly trade-offs.

Somewhere along the way, in my personal opinion, playing sport for the love of sport has been lost, from the demise of the sandlot to the commercialization of sports with multi-million-dollar athlete contracts. My grandfather played football in the late 1930s and the early 1940s, a time when none of us would have considered a helmet necessary. Those football players were paid a fraction of what athletes are paid today.

Sometimes they were paid just $10 or $20 a week, not $1 million a week. I question at times whether we're really better off today than we were all those years ago. Sport is certainly more exciting and flashier, with more glitz and glam, but what price have we paid?

How to Get the Same Level of Care as Professional Athletes

This book is for athletic trainers, coaches, and parents to act as a resource that they wouldn't normally have. If you have concerns about your child's health, if they have an injury you'd like examined, or you're wondering whether or not they may be susceptible to injury, you can also visit my website at **www.DrRobertBerry.com**, where there is a significant amount of support available.

My website has many great video resources. If you have an athlete about whom you're concerned, they would be evaluated by one of our sports-medicine specialists. They would go through a history and an exam and potentially advanced imaging to diagnose the problem. They would then have an accurate assessment of the problem, with a multi-faceted program and a plan to get them "back in the game." That may be physical therapy and working with certain bio-mechanic coaches in order to correct bio-mechanic problems that may have led to injuries. It might even include working with sports psychologists to address some of the anxiety or depression issues I wrote about. We would put together a comprehensive plan to help the athlete.

I am often asked what I do differently to take care of youthful "regular people" as opposed to professional athletes. The answer is: Nothing. Youth athletes can come and see someone who spent a good part of their career taking care of professional athletes, and they can get that same level of care. Visit **www.DrRoberyBerry.com**, or email us at **contactus@sportsmedtx.com** to get started.

www.ingramcontent.com/pod-product-compliance
Lightning Source LLC
Chambersburg PA
CBHW070102210526
45170CB00012B/715